The Mind and Body Massage

The Mind and Body Massage

The Guide to Ultimate Relaxation Uniting Massage, Music and Aroma Therapies

Cynthia S. Canaday

Writers Club Press
San Jose New York Lincoln Shanghai

The Mind and Body Massage
The Guide to Ultimate Relaxation Uniting Massage, Music and Aroma Therapies

All Rights Reserved © 2001 by Cynthia S. Canaday

No part of this book may be reproduced or transmitted in any form or by any means, graphic, electronic, or mechanical, including photocopying, recording, taping, or by any information storage or retrieval system, without the permission in writing from the publisher.

Writers Club Press
an imprint of iUniverse.com, Inc.

For information address:
iUniverse.com, Inc.
5220 S 16th, Ste. 200
Lincoln, NE 68512
www.iuniverse.com

ISBN: 0-595-17638-0

Printed in the United States of America

Contents

Preface ix

Introduction xi

Chapter 1 What You Will Need 3

Chapter 2 What To Do 11

Chapter 3 Massage Techniques 17

Chapter 4 The Massage 23

    1st Track   Celtic Sea–The Lats and Traps (5:56) 23

    2nd Track   Sheltered Shores–The Erector Bump
                    (one side) 5:40 26

    3rd Track   Highland Ascent–The Erector Bump
                    (other side) 5:57 28

    4th Track   Raging Sea–The Shoulder
                    (one side) 6:13 29

    5th Track   Thundering Gale–The Shoulder
                    (other side) 6:11 33

6th Track	Glenagriff Waters–The Neck and Scalp (6:02)	35
7th Track	Monk's Haven–The Legs and Glutes (5:57)	39
8th Track	Glenagriff Waters–The Foot (6:02)	42
9th Track	Sheltered Shores–The Other Foot (5:40)	44
10th Track	Celtic Sea—Total Body (5:56)	46

About the Author 49

Appendix The Mind and Body Massage 53

References 55

List of Illustrations

Latissimus Dorsi-outer back 25

Trapezius (Lower Fibers)-middle back 25

Erector Spinae 27, 37

Rhomboids 27, 30

Splenius 27, 37

Supraspinatus 30

Infraspinatus 30

Teres Major 31

Teres Minor 31

Trapezius (Upper Fibers) 32, 36

Levator Scapulae 32

Deltoid (Lateral) 32

Deltoid (Posterior) 32

Trapezius (Middle Fibers) 36

Sternocleidomastoid 38

Hamstrings 40

Gluteus Maximus 40

Gastrocnemius 41

Soleus 41

Preface

You could call this book "How to Give (or Receive) the Most Incredible Massage in the World" if you'd like.

After receiving professional massages regularly, my husband and I decided to try our hand at therapeutic home massage. After some training, we developed an environment and techniques for the most wonderful massage experience we have ever had.

Your senses will come alive…all of them. You will be transported to a third dimension where you will experience ocean waves crashing around you, a storm approaching and retreating, and finally nature returning to its serene state. Your olfactory sense will take in an aroma to lift you beyond that third dimension, and the relaxation your body achieves will be greater than anything you have ever imagined.

My husband and I were in Florida on vacation when we first enjoyed this experience. We had our massage table set up in our condo next to an open door where we could hear the sound of the surf, the seagulls, and all of the other majestic sounds of the sea. We had an aromatic massage oil to try, and that massage was the most extraordinary massage I had ever received. When we returned home, I was determined to duplicate that experience in the comfort of our in-town home. The results were astounding and even better than our vacation experience. I was then inspired to write this book to share our discovery with others.

Come journey with us, but be prepared. You will want to return often.

Introduction

It is no news that stress has a profound impact on both the mind and the body. Not only do we incur stress related to our jobs on a daily basis, but there is the stress associated with non work-related activities such as child rearing, providing for the family, death in the family, divorce, moving, financial difficulties, etc. The American Institute of Stress (AIS) is a non profit organization founded in 1978 to serve as a clearinghouse for information on all stress-related subjects. Its Board of Trustees is comprised of physicians and health professionals with expertise in various stress-related disorders. Some of their areas of expertise include cardiovascular disease, gastrointestinal and skin disease, immune system disturbances, thyroid disorders, and many viral-linked disorders ranging from herpes and the common cold to cancer and AIDS. The AIS states there is a growing confirmation that stress is a contributing factor in heart disease, hypertension, sudden death, depression, anxiety, smoking, obesity, alcoholism, substance abuse, cancer, arthritis, gastrointestinal and skin disorders, and a host of infections and immune system disorders.[1]

The AIS claims that stress is the number one health problem in the United States.[2] This claim is supported by these staggering facts:

- 43% of all adults suffer adverse health effects due to stress
- 75–90% of all visits to primary care physicians are for stress-related complaints or disorders
- Stress has been linked to all of the leading causes of death including heart disease, cancer, lung disease, accidents, cirrhosis and suicide
- Stress is said to be responsible for more than half of the 550,000,000 workdays lost annually because of absenteeism
- 60–80% of industrial accidents are due to stress
- Nine out of ten job stress lawsuits are successful with an average payout more than four times that for regular injury claims
- The market for stress management programs, products and services was approximately $11.31 billion for 1999, over a 20% increase from the 1995 market.

The number of stress-related websites on the Internet is astounding. In one query, the Lycos search engine returned 2,563,858 websites related to stress.

The Role of Massage Therapy in Relieving Stress

The survey of alternative medicine published in the January, 1993 edition of *The New England Journal of Medicine* ranked Massage Therapy third among the most frequently used forms of alternative health care. The key principles to any of the wide varieties of Massage Therapy are as follows:[3]

- ➢ Circulation of Blood
- ➢ Movement of Lymphatic Fluid
- ➢ Release of Toxins
- ➢ Release of Tension
- ➢ Interdependencies of Structure and Function
- ➢ Enhancement of All Bodily Systems
- ➢ Energy
- ➢ Mind / Body Integration, and
- ➢ **Reduction of Stress**

Massage therapy is an effective non-drug method for reducing stress and promoting relaxation. In addition to stress reduction, studies have documented benefits for amputations, arthritis, cerebral palsy, cerebral vascular accident, fibrositis syndrome, menstrual cramps, paraplegia/quadriplegia, scoliosis, acute and chronic pain, acute and chronic inflammation, chronic lymphedema, nausea, muscle spasm, soft tissue dysfunctions, grand mal epileptic seizures, anxiety, depression, insomnia, and psychoemotional stress which may aggravate significant mental illness.[3]

Prior to the advent of pharmaceutical medicine earlier in this century, references to massage therapy and research were not uncommon in mainstream medical literature. There were over six hundred articles in various journals such as the *Journal of the American Medical Association, British Medical Journal,* and others from 1813 to 1939. After World War I, there was a decline in focus on this field as drugs and other allopathic interventions gained the foreground. In the former Soviet countries, Germany, Japan and China, massage therapists still work alongside doctors as part of the healthcare team. Massage therapy is fully integrated into the healthcare system in China where hospitals have massage wards, and it is covered by national health insurance in Germany.[3]

Most insurance companies do not cover the cost of massage and bodywork in the United States; this cost is placed on the individual. Because of this high cost, home massage, as instructed in *The Mind and Body Massage,* is an excellent alternative to relieving stress and supporting healthy bodily function.

Massage therapy obviously has a very broad, diverse range of applications. It can support any health condition that would benefit from greater blood circulation and the release of tension.

Psychological conditions are also beneficially affected from massage, as the physiological changes that occur with this kind of intervention help harmonize and rebalance the nervous and hormonal systems.[3]

One of the previously stated key principles of massage therapy was Mind / Body Integration. As Dr. William Collinge, M.P.H., Ph.D. states, the "Mind and body have a reciprocal relationship. Soma (body) affects psyche (mind) and vice versa. Hence there can be somatopsychic effects, in which the conditions of the body affect the mind and emotions, and there can be psychosomatic effects, in which psychological or emotional conditions affect the body. Change in one domain may cause change in the other. Often psychotherapy and massage therapy or bodywork complement each other."[3]

As you may find, most books on massage currently in the marketplace concentrate on the physical aspects of massage but do not address the need to affect the mind. The calming effects of a mental journey provided in *The Mind and Body Massage* allow the mind to accomplish the same relaxation the body is achieving through physical manipulation.

Inclusion of Music Therapy

Music Therapy is defined as "The use of music by a qualified person to effect the positive changes in the psychological, physical, cognitive, or social functioning of individuals with health or educational problems."[4]

The idea of music as a healing influence which could affect health and behavior is as least as old as the writings of Aristotle and Plato. The 20th century discipline began after World War I and World War II when community musicians of all types, both amateur and professional, went to Veterans hospitals around the country to play for the thousands of veterans suffering both physical and emotional trauma from the wars. The patients' notable physical and emotional responses to music led the doctors and nurses to request the hiring of musicians by the hospitals.[4]

The benefits of Music Therapy in hospitals today are as follows:[4]

- Alleviate pain in conjunction with anesthesia or pain medication
- Elevate patients' mood and counteract depression
- Promote movement for physical rehabilitation
- Calm or sedate
- Help induce sleep

> Counteract apprehension or fear
> **Lessen muscle tension for the purpose of relaxation**

The American Music Therapy Association, founded in 1998 as a union of the National Association for Music Therapy and the American Association for Music Therapy, states that music therapy techniques can also be applied by healthy individuals for stress reduction. Active music making, such as drumming, as well as passive listening for relaxation are effective means for reducing stress.[4]

The nature recording used in *The Mind and Body Massage* provides the relaxation benefits suggested by the AMTA. It is a realistic combination of sounds from the sea, the sky, and the natural habitat of earth's creatures.

The Added Benefit of Aromatherapy

Aromatherapy is derived from two words: Aroma, meaning fragrance or smell, and therapy, meaning treatment. Aromatherapy is often defined as the practice of using naturally distilled essences of plants to promote the health and well-being of the body. It combines the soothing, healing touch of massage with the therapeutic properties of Essential Oils. Aromatherapy is a holistic treatment which can have a profound effect on the mind, body and emotions.[5]

Many of the oils used in Aromatherapy have a long history of therapeutic use. Aromatherapy was used by the most ancient civilizations and is reputed to be at least 6000 years old. It is widely thought that Aromatherapy began in Egypt. A medical papyri considered to date back to around 1555 BC contains remedies for all types of illnesses and the methods of application are similar to the ones used in Aromatherapy and Herbal medicine today.[5]

The Mind and Body Massage uses an aromatic massage oil to enhance the state of relaxation achieved from the combination of massage and music therapies.

Chapter 1

What You Will Need

Because this massage incorporates three types of natural healthcare–massage therapy, music therapy and aroma therapy, it will be different from any massage you have ever experienced. A realistic nature recording is played during the massage allowing the massage recipient to feel as though they are on site in the natural environment. Aromatic massage oil is used to promote and enhance relaxation as well as stimulate one of the strongest of the body senses–the sense of smell. Particular body parts are massaged during specified tracks of the nature recording (and with specified strokes) keeping in sync with the theme of the particular track.

I have chosen to tell a story as it relates to the nature recording. If desired, massage recipients can take the imaginary journey I have created while receiving the massage, or they can create their own odyssey associated with each track.

To fully enjoy your Mind and Body Massage, you will need the following items. I will discuss each of the items following the list:

1. Thickly padded massage table with face cradle or massage mat with face cradle
2. Roll-type pillow for foot elevation
3. Soft beach towel or other body-size towel, two soft handkerchiefs, and soft hand towel
4. Rough-textured towel that you do not mind being stained
5. A warm, comfortable room
6. Programmable CD player, preferably with additional surround-sound speakers
7. Northsound Music Group's *Celtic Landscapes* CD
8. Quality, aromatic massage oil
9. A glass of wine, or other optional relaxation aid
10. Loving hands

Massage Table

If you enjoy massage, you really should invest in a massage table. You can use a massage mat, but because they are placed on a bed or the floor, there are limitations to their use. Access to the person receiving the massage (hereafter referred to as the 'recipient') is restricted, or the person giving the massage (the 'provider') spends an inordinate amount of time on their knees. You can buy a massage table from a local retailer, mail order catalogs, or an Internet warehouse such as eBay. We purchased our custom-made table directly from a merchant on eBay and the transaction was painless. Our table was delivered to our door within a week's time. Make sure your table includes a face cradle to prevent neck strain and allow access to the muscles in the neck.

Roll-type Pillow

A roll-type pillow placed under the ankles alleviates pressure on the back, hips and knees. It also enables the provider to more easily massage the feet. If you do not have a roll-type pillow, you can use a regular bed pillow, folded in half lengthwise, for this purpose.

Linens

A soft beach towel, or other body-size towel, should be placed under the recipient to protect the table from oil and provide a layer of warmth between the recipient and the table. Two soft handkerchiefs should be positioned on the face cradle to prevent the facial skin from sticking to the cradle surface. A soft hand towel can be placed around the roll-type pillow to protect its fabric.

Rough-textured Towel

After the massage is completed, a rough-textured towel will be used to 'dry off' the recipient. Sesame oil is the primary ingredient in many massage oils, and this oil can stain fabrics as well as leave a lingering odor. Therefore, this should be a towel that you do not mind being soiled. I have found that Febreze Clean Wash Laundry Aid added to the wash helps to remove some of the odor that lingers on the linens.

Room Environment

Because massage is best enjoyed completely undressed, a warm, comfortable room is essential to the recipient's comfort. In addition, some massage oils contain herbal extracts that have a cooling effect on the skin. Therefore, the room temperature should compensate for the cooling sensation that might be experienced.

CD Player

To provide a one-hour massage and allow the recipient to mentally transcend from one nature environment to another during the experience, the CD player must be programmable. In addition, properly placed surround-sound speakers allow the recipient to be enveloped in the sound.

CD

Northsound Music Group's *Celtic Landscapes* CD is the best nature recording I have ever heard. It contains a multitude of sounds on the convenience of one CD and is the perfect recording for the journey the massage recipient will take during The Mind and Body Massage. You can buy *Celtic Landscapes* at your local bookstore or audio retailer, or you can order it directly from Northsound Music Group. Their website address is *www.northsoundmusic.com* or you can call them directly at 715 356-9800.

Massage Oil

A quality, aromatic massage oil will heighten the sense of smell while the mind is traveling through its journey and the body is achieving ultimate relaxation. Everyone has different fragrances they prefer, but three that I especially like are as follows:

❖ Elemis Aromapure 'Aching Muscle Massage Oil'® by Steiner Leisure Limited. This beautifully fragranced Sweet Almond oil also contains pure essential oils of Chamomile, Birch, Pine, Rosemary and Thyme. Although a bit expensive, I think it is well worth the extra cost.

❖ 'Romance' Aromathology Massage Oil® by Crabtree & Evelyn. This oil contains a blend of rose, sandalwood, ylang ylang and cardamom–essential oils known to enhance feelings of warmth and openness. 'Romance' is also available in 4 inch and 6 inch pillar candles to enhance the room's aroma.

❖ 'Stress Relief' Aromatherapy Massage Oil® by Bath & Body Works. This eucalyptus and spearmint oil is infused with St. John's Wort releasing a stress-relieving fragrance and helping to soothe skin.

All three of these oils have a clean and sensuous aroma. You can buy 'Romance' and 'Stress Relief' at your local Crabtree & Evelyn or Bath & Body Works retailer. You can buy the Elemis massage oil on-line at *www.timetospa.com*. 'Romance' is also available on-line at www.crabtree-evelyn.com.

Relaxation Aid

A relaxation aid is optional, of course, but my husband and I enjoy the added benefit that it provides.

The Hands

You do not have to have experience with massage to give (and receive) an incredible one. I will explain the techniques you will use and when you will use them. All that is required of you is a little study and the desire to please your partner. You will then reap the benefits in return!

Chapter 2

What To Do

To give (or receive) this massage experience, you will need to do the following:

Set Up the Massage Table

The massage table should be set up in a warm comfortable room, free from outside disturbances. The beach towel should be placed on the table, handkerchiefs placed on the face cradle, and the roll pillow, covered by a hand towel, should be placed near the foot of the table. You will need to coordinate the placement of the CD player and speakers with the table to achieve the sound quality desired.

Set Your Room Temperature

We have found that a room temperature between 76° and 80° during the summer and between 74° and 77° during the winter provides the warmth necessary for the massage. In addition, this allows the recipient to be transported to the tropics where they will begin their experience basking in the warm sun.

Position Your CD Player and Speakers

The CD player should be positioned where the massage provider can view the display indicating time related to each track. The main speakers should be placed slightly in front of the recipient's head, equal distance apart, while the additional surround-sound speakers should be place slightly behind the recipient's feet, equal distance apart.

Program the Playback of the CD

The *Celtic Landscapes* CD should be programmed in the following order:

Order	Name	Track Number	Length
1st track	Celtic Sea	5	5:56
2nd track	Sheltered Shores	2	5:40
3rd track	Highland Ascent	3	5:57
4th track	Raging Sea	7	6:13
5th track	Thundering Gale	4	6:11
6th track	Glenagriff Waters	8	6:02
7th track	Monk's Haven	1	5:57

8th track	Glenagriff Waters	8	6:02
9th track	Sheltered Shores	2	5:40
10th track	Celtic Sea	5	5:56

Warm the Massage Oil (if desired)

A few minutes prior to the massage, place the tightly closed bottle of oil in a sink full of hot tap water to warm. If you choose not to warm the oil with hot tap water, make sure you warm it in your hands prior to applying it to the recipient's body. Never pour cold oil directly onto the skin.

Enjoy Your Glass of Wine

Both the massage recipient and provider should enjoy the relaxation aid. In this case it is definitely as enjoyable to give as to receive!

Give the Massage

The recipient should lie face down on the table to prepare for the massage. Because comfort and relaxation is the ultimate goal in the massage, a towel or sheet may be placed over the recipient's rear if modesty and exposure is a concern. You can gently fold the sides of the towel or sheet in for working the glutes, but to help the recipient feel secure, be sure to fold them back down before proceeding to the next body part. In the following chapter, you will be instructed on massage techniques and be given guidelines to help you give the most relaxing massage conceivable. In the subsequent chapter, the recipient will be guided through their imaginary journey, while you are instructed on the specific massage techniques to use on the various parts of the body.

'Dry Off' the Recipient

After all tracks have been played and the massage is complete, take advantage of the silence to remove surface oil with the rough-textured towel. To provide a contrast to the massage, vary your strokes and technique. Because the recipient may feel a little light-headed after the massage, pay special attention to the feet to prevent injury when stepping off of the table.

Chapter 3

Massage Techniques

Massage is an ancient practice that increases the flow of oxygen and nutrients to the cells while helping to remove cell waste. When muscles are overworked, they tighten and restrict the flow of fluids through their fibers. This dehydration causes the muscle to constrict. The decrease in circulation can also cause cool spots to appear on the body. A healthy muscle is soft and fluid, not hard and lumpy. Massage gets the fluids flowing and returns the muscle to its healthy state.[6]

The Strokes

There are three basic strokes used in this massage. I will discuss each of these strokes and the application for them. Specific uses will be discussed in the next chapter.

Whole Hand Stroke

The whole hand stroke is achieved by molding the entire hand to the recipient's body. The stroke is performed using either a back and forth or circular motion and is best used on surface muscles to request access to underlying muscles.

Fingertip Stroke

The fingertip stroke is achieved by using the pads of the fingertips and extending the fingers in a rigid position from the hand. The idea is to massage using the muscles in the arm, not the hand or fingers. The fingers are an extension of the hand and the hand an extension of the arm. The arm, thus the fingers, are moved in a back and forth motion, and this stroke is used to massage underlying muscles where deeper penetration is required.

Thumb Stroke

Like the fingertip stroke, the thumb stroke is achieved by using the pads of the thumb and extending the thumb in a rigid position from the hand. Again, you are using the larger muscles in the arm with a back and forth motion preventing the smaller muscles in the thumb and hand from tiring. This stroke is used in conjunction with the fingertip stroke and is best when working the shoulders from the head of the table or the feet from the end of the table.

The Guidelines

There are several guidelines to help the massage recipient feel comfortable and secure under your hand and to prevent you from tiring during the process:[6]

1. Keep both hands on the body at all times. When you are massaging with one hand, rest the other hand on the body. You do not want the recipient to be wondering what you are doing with your other hand.

2. When working large areas such as the back or legs, share the work between your two hands. When you reach the mid-part of your body with one hand, switch to the resting hand to prevent muscles from tiring.

3. Feel for cold spots indicating lack of circulation, not just lumpy muscles.

4. Use lots of oil to prevent friction from building up between the recipient's skin and your hands.

5. Massage should be firm, but not painful. Ask the recipient to let you know if the stroke is too firm or not firm enough. Otherwise, dialogue during the massage could be counter-productive to the relaxation you are trying to achieve.

6. Use your body to leverage your strokes.

7. When working from the side of the table, unless otherwise instructed, work the side of the body closest to you.

8. When working the back, work from the base of the spine (the sacrum) towards the neck. When you reach the neck, transition your hands back to the sacrum and start over. Do not massage down the back.

9. Pay attention to the time remaining on the CD display. To prevent an abrupt change of body location, begin transitioning your hands to the next body part during the last 5-10 seconds of a particular track.

10. Because muscles release toxins into the body during a massage, the recipient should drink plenty of water the following 24 hours to rid the body of toxic waste.

The Program

In the following chapter, I will specify the part of the body to massage with each track from the CD and indicate the specific massage technique that should be used on that body part. The Appendix contains a page that can be detached and used as a reference while you are giving the massage. Times for each track are indicated on this page allowing you to transition to the next body part prior to the end of the track. The reference page also contains the body part to work during a particular track.

Chapter 4

The Massage

1ˢᵗ Track   *Celtic Sea–The Lats and Traps (5:56)*

It is a beautiful, warm, sunny day–not a cloud in the sky. You are basking in the tropical sun, and you can almost feel the surf splashing on your face. The white, sandy beach goes on for miles and miles, and you are alone with the wonders of nature. Waves are crashing onto the shore where the sandpipers are running frantically as if trying not to get their feet wet. The seagulls are flying overhead and you spot a pelican diving for its meal. You watch two dolphins jumping in the distance and marvel at their grace. A conch shell has washed up on the shore, and you remember the almost ghostly sound it makes when blown. Gazing towards the heavens you see the great palm trees swaying in the slight breeze that brushes lightly over your skin. Resting your head, you can almost feel the waves roll through you as they approach from the west, pass in front of you, and trail off to the east. The water then ebbs back to create another wave that almost takes you with it. The wave patterns are hypnotizing as you fall into a deep state of relaxation.

###############

As the journey begins for the massage recipient, you will begin the massage. Start by applying plenty of warm oil to the entire back–from the hips, up the back, and down the arms to the elbows. Eventually position yourself at your partner's head and beginning at the shoulders, use both hands to stroke down the back near the spine, up the outer edges of the back, and off of the arms. Repeat this movement as you feel the tides take over your body as well. After approximately three minutes, move to one side of the table, and working the opposite side of the body, use the whole hand stroke, molding your hands to your partner's body to gently massage the outer back (Latissimus Dorsi) and the lower fibers of the Trapezius comprising the middle back. When there is about a minute and a half left on the track, move to the other side of the table and repeat the whole hand stroke on the opposite side of the body. Remember to keep one hand on your partner at all times.

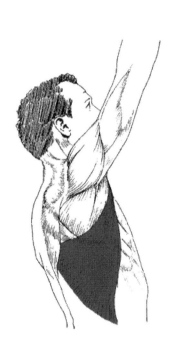
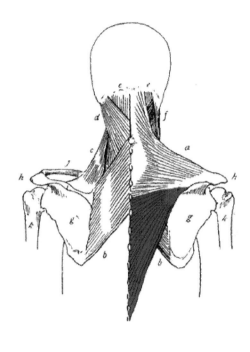

Latissimus Dorsi-outer back   *Trapezius (Lower Fibers)-middle back*

2nd Track   Sheltered Shores–The Erector Bump (one side) 5:40

The air is becoming still; the waves have subsided into mere lapping on the shore. The breeze is building, but there is a strange calm in the air. The seagulls seem to be preparing for something, but you are not sure for what. You observe a sea turtle slowing moving away from the water's edge heading for its nest. A crab emerges from one of the waves, quickly runs sideways and buries itself in the sand. Soon the pelicans, sandpipers and other birds join the gulls in their preparation. The wind is starting to pick up from the west. You lie in your tranquil state. Nothing can harm you from where you are.

###############

The Erector Spinae muscles lie along both sides of the spine. They run under the Rhomboids in the middle of the back as well as the neck extensors (Splenius) and surface again at the base of the skull.

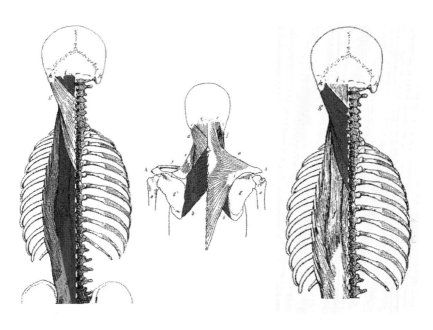

Erector Spinae   *Rhomboids*   *Splenius*

During this track, you will position yourself at the side of the table. Working the opposite side of the body and starting at the base of the spine (sacrum), use the fingertip stroke and move your hand back and forth across the erector, gradually moving towards the neck. Remember to keep both hands on your partner, and switch hands when you approach the center of your body. Once you reach the shoulders, transition your hand back to the sacrum and start over. Do not massage down the back with this stroke. The neck portion of the erector will be massaged at a later time. The erector muscles feel like a tight rope surrounding the spine. This is a very effective stroke for loosening that rope-like muscle to produce fluidity.

3rd Track   Highland Ascent–The Erector Bump (other side) 5:57

The water has an eerie calm as the wind picks up. The birds are preparing their brood to seek shelter. You hear thunder in the distance; then it subsides. A strange silence fills the air, but the wind swirlling around you announces the storm that is quickly approaching. You let the wind lift you up where you are safe and can watch the storm below.

##############

Move to the other side of the table where you will work the opposite side of the body. Again, using the fingertip stroke, start at the base of the spine and work your way towards the neck, moving back and forth across the erector, switching hands at the center of your body. Remember to keep your fingers extended and use your body to leverage your arm strokes. Once you reach the shoulders, transition your hand back to the sacrum and start over. Do not massage down the back with this stroke. The neck portion of the erector will be massaged at a later time.

4th Track Raging Sea–The Shoulder *(one side) 6:13*

From your perch high above the clouds, you hear the loud clap of thunder and the rolling sound it makes as it fades into the distance. You remember being a small child and thinking thunder sounded like the angels were bowling. You smile remembering how safe you felt under your covers when you notice the waves have picked back up and changed direction. The thunder moves closer as lightening strikes on the horizon. The tides are high, and there are no signs of the seagulls or pelicans as they have sought shelter. You see ships swaying back and forth trying to return to port. You are not worried….the wind is your companion.

###############

The shoulder is comprised of many muscles, some surrounding the shoulder blades known as rotator cuff muscles (the Supraspinatus, the Infraspinatus, the Teres Major and the Teres Minor). Others make up the upper shoulder muscles that are responsible for lifting the shoulders (the upper fibers of the Trapezius and the Levator Scapulae), while still others are located on the side of the shoulders going down the arm (the Deltoids). This group of muscles is responsible for most stress that individuals feel in their bodies.

The massage of these muscles will be performed both at the side of the table and at the recipient's head. Start at the side of the table near one shoulder. Using the fingertip stroke, begin with the portion of the Rhomboids closest to the triangular shaped scapula (shoulder blade). Gradually work your way around the scapula. You will feel the Supraspinatus near the top of the scapula, the Infraspinatus directly on top of the scapula, and the the Teres Major and Teres Minor below the scapula. Use caution when massaging these muscles and do not exert too much pressure on them.

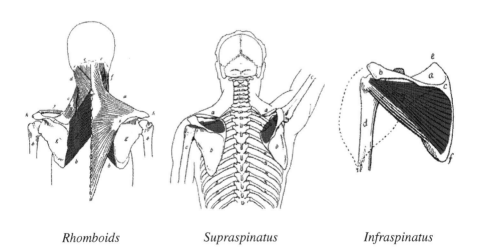

Rhomboids *Supraspinatus* *Infraspinatus*

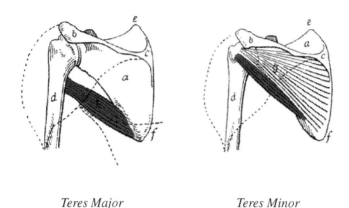

Teres Major   *Teres Minor*

After approximately 2-1/2 minutes, move to the head of the table. Using the thumb stroke, begin massaging the upper fibers of the Trapezius, a surface muscle, on the same side of the body. You should then be able to reach the Levator Scapulae underneath (the stress muscle), and work from the shoulder blade towards the neck with the same thumb stroke. Alternately work the deltoids (both lateral and posterior) until the end of the track.

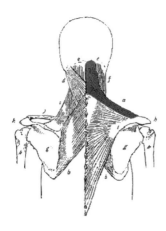
Trapezius (Upper Fibers)

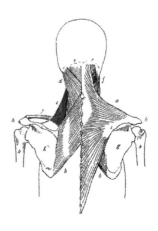
Levator Scapulae

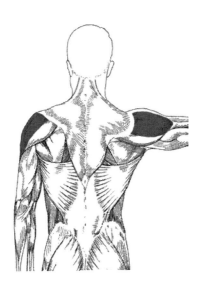
Deltoid (Lateral)

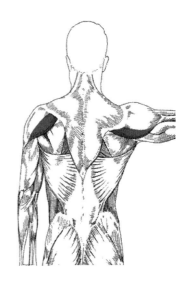
Deltoid (Posterior)

5th Track   Thundering Gale–The Shoulder (other side) 6:11

The rain has begun. Its steady rhythm almost puts you to sleep. The wind is such a soft mattress; you wonder if you can stay here forever. The rain pounds harder below you as the silence grows. You watch a single raindrop as it descends and disappears into the ocean. You wonder if life under the sea even knows that it is raining. You smell the air–a distinct redolence that can only be the rain. Finally the storm moves to the east, but you can still hear the distant rumbling of thunder in the distance. You are sad in a way…you love the cleansing rain…and your protector the wind.

###############

As you move to the opposite side of the table to work the other shoulder, position your fingertips on the portion of the Rhomboids closest to the scapula. After working the Rhomboids, gradually work your way around the scapula gently massaging the four rotator cuff muscles. After approximately 2-1/2 minutes, once again move to the head of the table. Using the thumb stroke, begin massaging the two upper shoulder muscles on the same side of the body. Alternately work both the lateral and posterior deltoids until the end of the track. Remember to keep your thumb extended and use the larger muscles in your arm to perform the massage.

6th Track   Glenagriff Waters–The Neck and Scalp (6:02)

The rain has subsided. The wind gently transports you to an open meadow and places you beside a stream which is now flowing hard because of the rain. Birds you have never seen before suddenly surround you to welcome you to their home. An owl even joins in the greeting. Fish, now abundant in the stream, are searching for food stirred up from the storm. The sun is trying to peep its way through the clouds, but can't quite make its way through the pillowy masses. You stare at the clouds and try to make out images. You drop your eyes and realize you have never seen grass so green. It must be the tears in your eyes as the wind waves farewell.

###############

Because gravity constantly pushes the head into the spine, neck compression results. One purpose of the neck massage is to create length in the neck so that the underlying erector muscles feathering up into the cranium can be worked.

Position yourself at the head of the table. Using the fingers of both hands, massage the upper and middle fibers of the Trapezius by creating a pulling motion from each shoulder up to the top of the neck and also from the center of the back to the top of the neck. Repeat this stretching stroke several times.

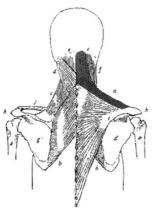

Trapezius (Upper Fibers)   *Trapezius (Middle Fibers)*

Once the Trapezius has been stretched, use the thumb stroke to bump the upper portion of the erectors away from the spine. Repeat the combination of stretch and massage, stretch and massage until the muscles feel soft and fluid. You will also be working the Splenius muscle positioned diagonally on the neck during this time.

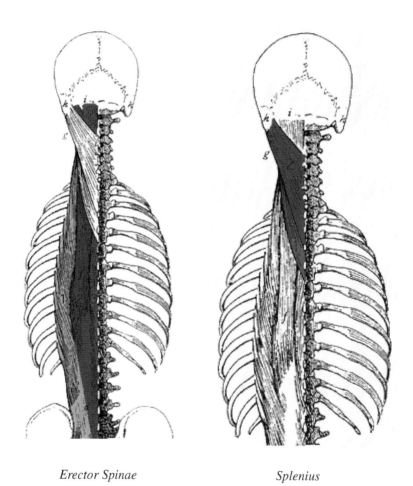

Erector Spinae   *Splenius*

The Sternocleidomastoid muscles are located on the side of the neck. Using two fingers on each hand, gently massage these muscles by motioning your hand up and down (from the back of the neck towards the front) while you move from the base of the neck towards the skull.

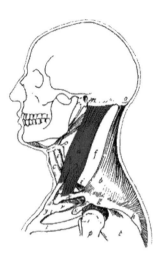

Sternocleidomastoid

Next, curl your fingers in a clawing position and place your fingers at the base of the scalp. Using a circular motion, slowly move your way up the back of the head massaging the scalp.

7th Track Monk's Haven–The Legs and Glutes (5:57)

You are transported to a steamy cove where previously dried-up waterfalls are now flowing slightly because of the rain. You don't know how you got there, but it doesn't matter—the steady stream of water into the pool calms your mind. You can see your reflection in the pool when you notice a tiny frog gazing up at you from under a rock. Startled, you lift your eyes to the sky to see birds with magnificent colors shaking their feathers and spreading their wings, feeling glorious after nature's bath.

###############

You will work three primary muscle groups during this track: the Hamstrings, the Calf and the Glutes. Position yourself at one side of the table. Working the leg immediately in front of you and using the whole hand and thumb stroke, begin massaging the Hamstrings with long strokes going from the back of the knee up to the rear. When you reach the rear, use the palm of your hand to work the Gluteus Maximus located on the side of the rear. Since both the Hamstrings and the Gluteus Maximus are large muscles, use long, big strokes to massage them, but be gentle if necessary to prevent bruising.

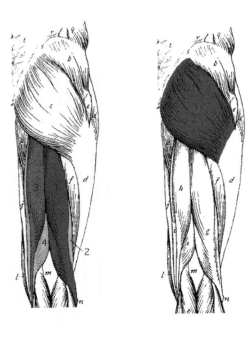

Hamstrings *Gluteus Maximus*

There are two primary muscles comprising the calf: the Gastrocnemius and the Soleus. Work these muscles in the same way as the Hamstrings and the Glutes–with long strokes using the whole hand and the thumb. Moving down the calf towards the ankle, massage the Achilles as well.

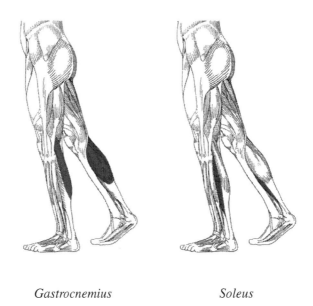

Gastrocnemius   *Soleus*

After about 3 minutes, move to the other side of the table (keeping a hand on your partner as you move) and work the other leg.

8th Track   Glenagriff Waters–The Foot (6:02)

The sun is now shining brightly as one of its rays gently picks you up and lays you down beside a babbling brook flowing into the ocean. You listen to the sounds of wildlife blissful that the skies have cleared and nature has returned to its serene state. You drink from the fresh water and wonder where the ocean accepts this small addition to its great mass. You begin to follow the stream in the direction the water flows. The birds lead the way, joyous that you have joined them for a brief moment in time.

###############

As with the hands, there are many, many muscles in the feet. Therefore, you are going to concentrate on primary areas instead. Position yourself at the foot of the table. Hold the front of the foot with one hand and use the thumb stroke to work the ball of the foot and the arch. Stretch out each toe by gently pushing from the base to the tip with your thumb. Do not work your fingers between the toes. Work the heel by firmly pressing from the back of the arch up over the heel. Squeeze the heel from the sides and repeat all strokes.

After about 3 minutes, lift the foot off the roll pillow and moving to the side of the table, bend the knee at a 90° angle so the foot is straight up in the air. Use your hands to flex and point the foot and rotate the ankle. Continue massaging the ball, arch and heel in this position. At the end of the track, rest the ankle back on the roll pillow.

9th Track   Sheltered Shores–The Other Foot (5:40)

Your journey down the stream leads you to a cove sheltered on three sides by rock walls. The wildlife thrives in the tranquility and you notice an insect buzzing. They are protected from birds in this haven. A breeze blows around the rock walls as the sun tries to break through the trees hanging overhead. You walk in the lapping surf and follow the shoreline out of the cove into the bright sunshine.

###############

Position yourself back at the foot of the table and work the opposite foot from that previously worked. Hold the front of the foot with one hand and use the thumb stroke to work the ball of the foot and the arch. Stretch out each toe by gently pushing from the base to the tip with your thumb. Do not work your fingers between the toes. Work the heel by firmly pressing from the back of the arch up over the heel. Squeeze the heel from the sides and repeat all strokes.

After about 3 minutes, lift the foot off the roll pillow and moving to the side of the table, bend the knee at a 90° angle so the foot is straight up in the air. Use your hands to flex and point the foot and rotate the ankle. Continue massaging the ball, arch and heel in this position. At the end of the track, rest the ankle back on the roll pillow.

10th Track   Celtic Sea—Total Body (5:56)

You wander down the shoreline until you see the familiar white sandy beach from where your journey began. The ocean swells have resumed and the seagulls have returned overhead. A long-legged blue heron is casually strolling along the water's edge. You feel the cool, wet sand squish between your toes as you lift the conch shell washed up before the storm. Putting it to your ear, you hear the roar of the ocean within. You take in the smell of the salt air, the warmth of the sun and the slight breeze as you lie down beside the surf as your journey ends.

##############

Use this track to cover all areas of the body previous massaged separately. Position yourself on one side of the table at the recipient's hips. Use the whole hand to work the side of the body closest to you. Move one hand from the rear, down the leg, and to the feet while the other hand moves up the back and off of the shoulders. Repeat this stroke several times with medium pressure, only moving hands in the opposite direction to re-position. Your partner should feel any negative energy exiting the body from the feet and shoulders with this stroke. Move to the opposite side of the table and repeat the stroke on the other leg and other side of the back.

Move to the head of the table and repeat the sweeping stroke done in the first track to spread the oil, except this time add the arms, shoulders and neck. Beginning at the base of the neck, use both hands to stroke down the back near the spine, up the outer edges of the back, down the backside of the arms, up the front side of the arms, across the upper shoulders and up the neck. The recipient should allow any negativity remaining to exit the body from the head with this final stroke.

For the last minute of the massage, use your nails (if neatly trimmed) to gently scratch your partner's back. Use long strokes as well as circular motions, and then be proud of the job you have done. You have just given your partner the best massage imaginable!

Take turns and enjoy!

About the Author

Ms. Canaday grew up in Birmingham, Alabama and graduated from Auburn University in 1978 with a Bachelor of Science in Business Administration (Accounting). Prior to attending college, she worked as a dance instructor for a local dance academy and was asked to choreograph dance performances for social organizations to which she belonged. She started her professional career as an auditor where writing audit reports was one of her primary responsibilities. After specializing in audits of the Information Technology function of a Fortune 500 company headquartered in Birmingham, she moved into the IT department where technical writing was one of her principal duties. She developed written control procedures over program development and installation activities and developed documentation standards and user-interface standards for legacy systems. She created user and technical reference manuals for the company's computer applications. She designed the data security system contained within those applications and developed a written corporate policy on data security. Because of her knowledge and excellent writing skills, she was asked to prepare written responses to external audit reports addressing weaknesses in control. She supervised contract personnel assisting in documentation preparation and introduced the need for quality assurance testing in the software release process. She was promoted to supervisor of the Systems Support function where she trained and supervised staff responsible for technical writing, quality assurance, data security, training, and user liaison activities. She was responsible for the Corporate Information Services Co-op Program where she recruited at college campuses and extended offers for employment. She planned work placement based on personal skill sets and department needs while acting as counselor/coach/motivator as needed.

She was a project leader for the company's Year 2000 project where she jointly developed the company's Y2K project strategy and managed the project management responsibilities for three of the company's divisions. She developed and held training sessions for twenty-three corporate departments and managed Y2K inventory files for the corporate office containing approximately 5000 hardware and software records.

Prior to her retirement in April, 2000 she was a member of the Sales Force Automation software selection team where one of her primary duties was to evaluate the adequacy of written documentation associated with the software.

She became interested in massage as a way to relieve the stress associated with her demanding career. She studied the art and techniques associated with massage and used her experience as a dancer to 'choreograph' the massage performed in this book. Her combination of artistic talent, creativity, and technical writing skills came together beautifully in the creation of her first book–*The Mind and Body Massage*.

Appendix

The Mind and Body Massage

Track	Track Length	Body Part
1st track (Celtic Sea)	5:56	The Lats and Traps
2nd track (Sheltered Shores)	5:40	The Erector (one side)
3rd track (Highland Ascent)	5:57	The Erector (other side)
4th track (Raging Sea)	6:13	The Shoulder (one side)
5th track (Thundering Gale)	6:11	The Shoulder (other side)
6th track (Glenagriff Waters)	6:02	The Neck and Scalp
7th track (Monk's Haven)	5:57	The Legs and Glutes
8th track (Glenagriff Waters)	6:02	The Foot
9th track (Sheltered Shores)	5:40	The Other Foot
10th track (Celtic Sea)	5:56	Total body

(Pull out for reference use)

References

1. The American Institute of Stress. *http://www.stress.org*
2. The American Institute of Stress. *Stress–America's #1 Health Problem. http://www.stress.org/problem.htm*
3. William Collinge, M.P.H., Ph.D. 1996. *Massage Therapy and Bodywork: Healing Through Touch.* Healthworld Online *http://www.healthy.net/library/books/search/bbody%5Fs.htm*
4. The American Music Therapy Association. *Frequently Asked Questions About Music Therapy. http://www.music-therapy.org/faqs.html*
5. The Kevala Centre. *Aromatherapy Origins and Background. http://www.kevala.co.uk/aromatherapy/introduction.htm*
6. 'Home Massage Instruction Video', an A2Z Possibilities, Inc. production featuring Will Green, President of the International Massage Association.
7. Muscle illustrations courtesy of James Griffing, M.S., B.S. and ExRx Online at *http://www.planetkc.com/exrx/Home.html*

Printed in Poland
by Amazon Fulfillment
Poland Sp. z o.o., Wrocław